This Journal Belongs To:

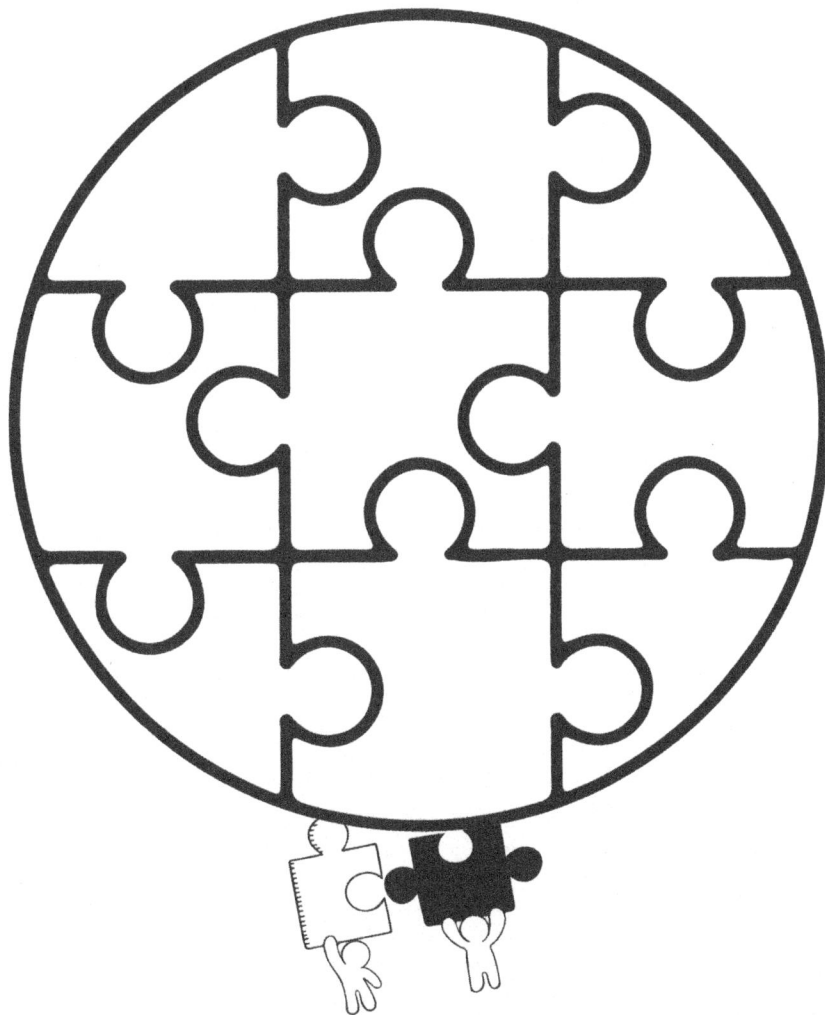

_____

PRIMARY GOALS

SPEECH & COMMUNICATION GOALS

SOCIAL SKILLS GOALS

SENSORY GOALS

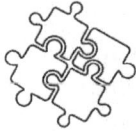 # ACTIVITY IDEAS

FINE MOTOR ACTIVITIES

VESTIBULAR/PROPRIOCEPTIVE

TACTILE

VISUAL

AUDITORY

ORAL

NOTES:

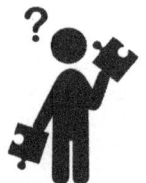

MILESTONE TRACKER

DATE:

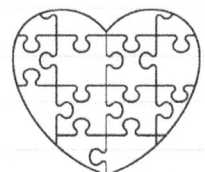

BOOKS TO READ

BOOK TITLE	✓	BOOK TITLE	✓

WEEK 1 ACTIVITIES:

MONDAY

TUESDAY

WEDNESDAY

THURSDAY

FRIDAY

SATURDAY

SUNDAY

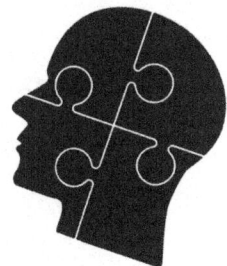

WEEK 1:

WEEK OF: _____

GOALS & PROGRESS
TRACKER

SPEECH & COMMUNICATION

SENSORY & O.T.

VESTIBULAR

TACTILE

ORAL MOTOR

MON

TUE

WED

THUR

FRI

SAT

SUN

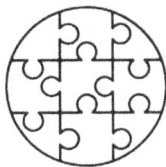

WEEK 1:

FINE MOTOR

VISUAL

AUDITORY

THIS WEEK'S CHALLENGES

THIS WEEK'S HIGHLIGHTS

SOCIAL SKILLS

FAVORITE MOMENT

WEEKLY APPOINTMENTS

WEEK OF:

MON

TUE

WED

THU

WEEKLY APPOINTMENTS

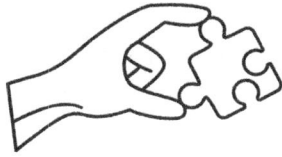

WEEK OF:

FRI

SAT

SUN

NOTES:

WEEKLY REFLECTION

Weekly Challenges

Weekly Accomplishments

Grateful For:

NOTES

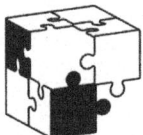

WEEK 2 ACTIVITIES:

MONDAY

TUESDAY

WEDNESDAY

THURSDAY

FRIDAY

SATURDAY

SUNDAY

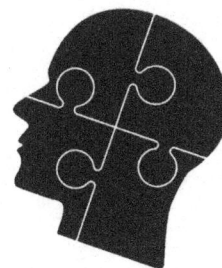

WEEK 2:

WEEK OF:

SPEECH & COMMUNICATION

SENSORY & O.T.

VESTIBULAR

TACTILE

ORAL MOTOR

MON

TUE

WED

THUR

FRI

SAT

SUN

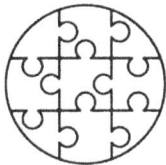

WEEK 2:

FINE MOTOR

VISUAL

AUDITORY

THIS WEEK'S CHALLENGES

SOCIAL SKILLS

THIS WEEK'S HIGHLIGHTS

FAVORITE MOMENT

WEEKLY APPOINTMENTS

WEEK OF:

_____

MON

_____
_____
_____
_____
_____

TUE

_____
_____
_____
_____
_____

WED

_____
_____
_____
_____
_____

THU

_____
_____
_____
_____
_____

WEEKLY APPOINTMENTS

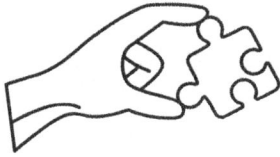

WEEK OF:

FRI

SAT

SUN

NOTES:

WEEKLY REFLECTION

Weekly Challenges

Weekly Accomplishments

Grateful For:

NOTES

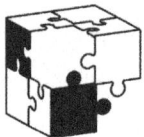

WEEK 3 ACTIVITIES:

MONDAY

TUESDAY

WEDNESDAY

THURSDAY

FRIDAY

SATURDAY

SUNDAY

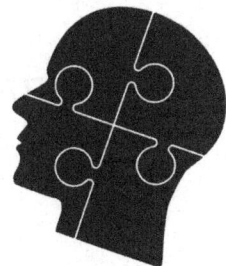

WEEK 3:

WEEK OF: _____

SPEECH & COMMUNICATION

SENSORY & O.T.

VESTIBULAR

TACTILE

ORAL MOTOR

MON

TUE

WED

THUR

FRI

SAT

SUN

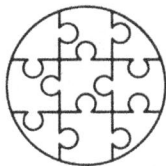

WEEK 3:

FINE MOTOR

VISUAL

AUDITORY

THIS WEEK'S CHALLENGES

THIS WEEK'S HIGHLIGHTS

SOCIAL SKILLS

FAVORITE MOMENT

WEEKLY APPOINTMENTS

WEEK OF:

MON

TUE

WED

THU

WEEKLY APPOINTMENTS

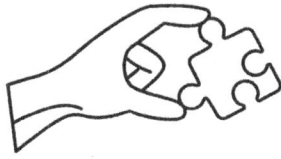

WEEK OF:

FRI

SAT

SUN

NOTES:

WEEKLY REFLECTION

Weekly Challenges

Weekly Accomplishments

Grateful For:

NOTES

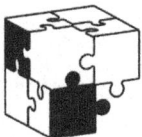

WEEK 4 ACTIVITIES:

MONDAY

TUESDAY

WEDNESDAY

THURSDAY

FRIDAY

SATURDAY

SUNDAY

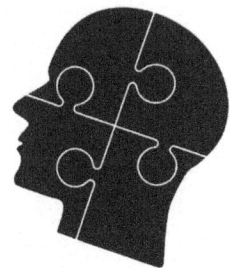

WEEK 4:

WEEK OF: _____

SPEECH & COMMUNICATION

SENSORY & O.T.

VESTIBULAR

TACTILE

ORAL MOTOR

MON

TUE

WED

THUR

FRI

SAT

SUN

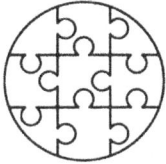

WEEK 4:

FINE MOTOR

VISUAL

AUDITORY

THIS WEEK'S CHALLENGES

THIS WEEK'S HIGHLIGHTS

SOCIAL SKILLS

FAVORITE MOMENT

WEEKLY APPOINTMENTS

WEEK OF:

MON

TUE

WED

THU

WEEKLY APPOINTMENTS

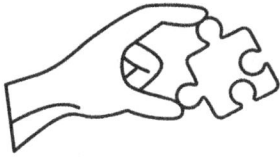

WEEK OF:

FRI

SAT

SUN

NOTES:

WEEKLY REFLECTION

Weekly Challenges

Weekly Accomplishments

Grateful For:

NOTES

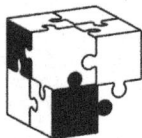

WEEK 5 ACTIVITIES:

MONDAY

TUESDAY

WEDNESDAY

THURSDAY

FRIDAY

SATURDAY

SUNDAY

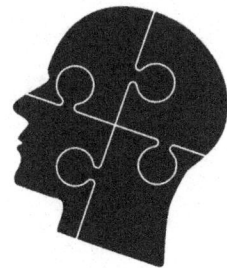

WEEK 5:

WEEK OF: _____

SPEECH & COMMUNICATION

SENSORY & O.T.

VESTIBULAR

TACTILE

ORAL MOTOR

MON

TUE

WED

THUR

FRI

SAT

SUN

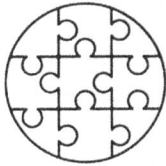

WEEK 5:

FINE MOTOR

VISUAL

AUDITORY

THIS WEEK'S CHALLENGES

THIS WEEK'S HIGHLIGHTS

SOCIAL SKILLS

FAVORITE MOMENT

WEEKLY APPOINTMENTS

WEEK OF:

MON

TUE

WED

THU

WEEKLY APPOINTMENTS

WEEK OF:

FRI

SAT

SUN

NOTES:

WEEKLY REFLECTION

Weekly Challenges

Weekly Accomplishments

Grateful For:

NOTES

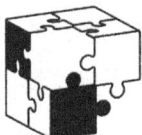

WEEK 6 ACTIVITIES:

MONDAY

TUESDAY

WEDNESDAY

THURSDAY

FRIDAY

SATURDAY

SUNDAY

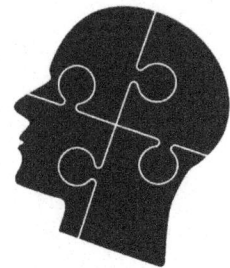

WEEK 6:

GOALS & PROGRESS
TRACKER

WEEK OF: _____

SPEECH & COMMUNICATION

SENSORY & O.T.

VESTIBULAR

TACTILE

ORAL MOTOR

MON

TUE

WED

THUR

FRI

SAT

SUN

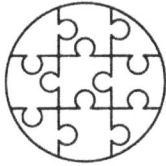

WEEK 6:

FINE MOTOR

VISUAL

AUDITORY

THIS WEEK'S CHALLENGES

SOCIAL SKILLS

THIS WEEK'S HIGHLIGHTS

FAVORITE MOMENT

WEEKLY APPOINTMENTS

WEEK OF:

_____

MON

_____
_____
_____
_____
_____

TUE

_____
_____
_____
_____
_____

WED

_____
_____
_____
_____
_____

THU

_____
_____
_____
_____

WEEKLY APPOINTMENTS

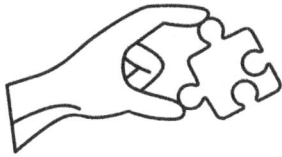

WEEK OF:

FRI

SAT

SUN

NOTES:

WEEKLY REFLECTION

Weekly Challenges

Weekly Accomplishments

Grateful For:

NOTES

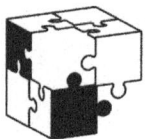

WEEK 7 ACTIVITIES:

MONDAY

TUESDAY

WEDNESDAY

THURSDAY

FRIDAY

SATURDAY

SUNDAY

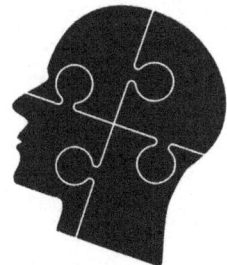

WEEK 7:

WEEK OF: _____

SPEECH & COMMUNICATION

SENSORY & O.T.

VESTIBULAR

TACTILE

ORAL MOTOR

MON

TUE

WED

THUR

FRI

SAT

SUN

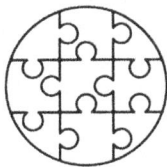

WEEK 7:

FINE MOTOR

VISUAL

AUDITORY

THIS WEEK'S CHALLENGES

THIS WEEK'S HIGHLIGHTS

SOCIAL SKILLS

FAVORITE MOMENT

WEEKLY APPOINTMENTS

WEEK OF:

MON

TUE

WED

THU

WEEKLY APPOINTMENTS

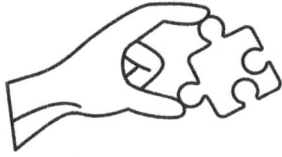

WEEK OF:

FRI

SAT

SUN

NOTES:

WEEKLY REFLECTION

Weekly Challenges

Weekly Accomplishments

Grateful For:

NOTES

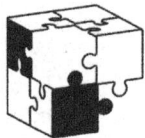

WEEK 8 ACTIVITIES:

MONDAY

TUESDAY

WEDNESDAY

THURSDAY

FRIDAY

SATURDAY

SUNDAY

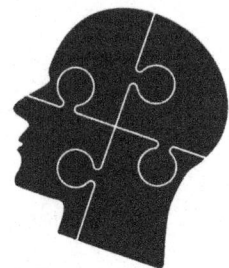

WEEK 8:

WEEK OF: _____

SPEECH & COMMUNICATION

SENSORY & O.T.

VESTIBULAR

TACTILE

ORAL MOTOR

MON

TUE

WED

THUR

FRI

SAT

SUN

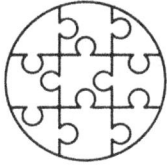

WEEK 8:

FINE MOTOR

VISUAL

AUDITORY

THIS WEEK'S CHALLENGES

THIS WEEK'S HIGHLIGHTS

SOCIAL SKILLS

FAVORITE MOMENT

WEEKLY APPOINTMENTS

WEEK OF:

MON

TUE

WED

THU

WEEKLY APPOINTMENTS

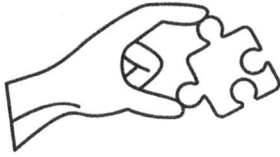

WEEK OF:

FRI

SAT

SUN

NOTES:

WEEKLY REFLECTION

Weekly Challenges

Weekly Accomplishments

Grateful For:

NOTES

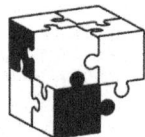

WEEK 9 ACTIVITIES:

MONDAY

TUESDAY

WEDNESDAY

THURSDAY

FRIDAY

SATURDAY

SUNDAY

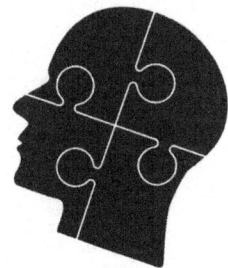

WEEK 9:

WEEK OF: _____

SPEECH & COMMUNICATION

SENSORY & O.T.

VESTIBULAR

TACTILE

ORAL MOTOR

MON

TUE

WED

THUR

FRI

SAT

SUN

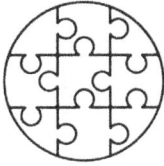

WEEK 9:

GOALS & PROGRESS
TRACKER

FINE MOTOR

VISUAL

AUDITORY

THIS WEEK'S CHALLENGES

THIS WEEK'S HIGHLIGHTS

SOCIAL SKILLS

FAVORITE MOMENT

WEEKLY APPOINTMENTS

WEEK OF:

MON

TUE

WED

THU

WEEKLY APPOINTMENTS

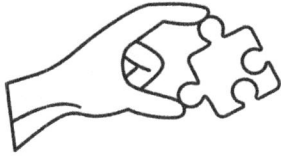

WEEK OF:

FRI

SAT

SUN

NOTES:

WEEKLY REFLECTION

Weekly Challenges

Weekly Accomplishments

Grateful For:

NOTES

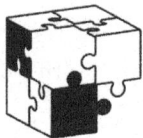

WEEK 10 ACTIVITIES:

MONDAY

TUESDAY

WEDNESDAY

THURSDAY

FRIDAY

SATURDAY

SUNDAY

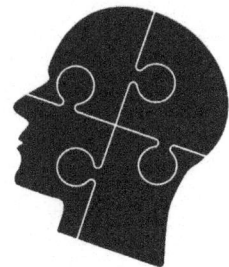

WEEK 10:

WEEK OF: _____

SPEECH & COMMUNICATION

SENSORY & O.T.

VESTIBULAR

TACTILE

ORAL MOTOR

MON

TUE

WED

THUR

FRI

SAT

SUN

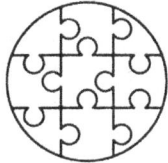

WEEK 10:

GOALS & PROGRESS
TRACKER

FINE MOTOR

VISUAL

AUDITORY

THIS WEEK'S CHALLENGES

SOCIAL SKILLS

THIS WEEK'S HIGHLIGHTS

FAVORITE MOMENT

WEEKLY APPOINTMENTS

WEEK OF:

MON

TUE

WED

THU

WEEKLY APPOINTMENTS

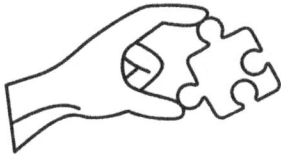

WEEK OF:

FRI

SAT

SUN

NOTES:

WEEKLY REFLECTION

Weekly Challenges

Weekly Accomplishments

Grateful For:

NOTES

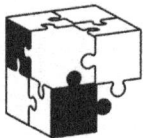

WEEK 11 ACTIVITIES:

MONDAY

TUESDAY

WEDNESDAY

THURSDAY

FRIDAY

SATURDAY

SUNDAY

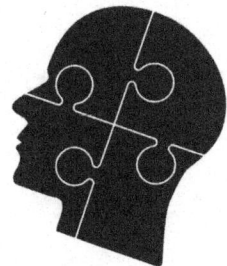

WEEK 11:

WEEK OF: _____

SPEECH & COMMUNICATION

SENSORY & O.T.

VESTIBULAR

TACTILE

ORAL MOTOR

MON

TUE

WED

THUR

FRI

SAT

SUN

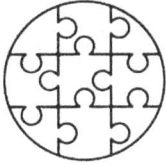

WEEK 11:

TRACKER

FINE MOTOR

VISUAL

AUDITORY

THIS WEEK'S CHALLENGES

THIS WEEK'S HIGHLIGHTS

SOCIAL SKILLS

FAVORITE MOMENT

WEEKLY APPOINTMENTS

WEEK OF:

MON

TUE

WED

THU

WEEKLY APPOINTMENTS

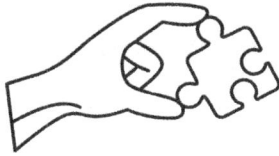

WEEK OF:

FRI

SAT

SUN

NOTES:

WEEKLY REFLECTION

Weekly Challenges

Weekly Accomplishments

Grateful For:

NOTES

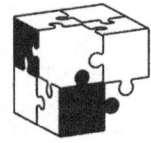

WEEK 12 ACTIVITIES:

MONDAY

TUESDAY

WEDNESDAY

THURSDAY

FRIDAY

SATURDAY

SUNDAY

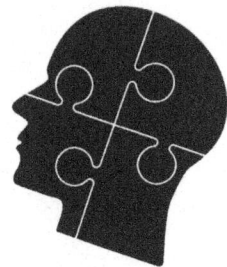

WEEK 12:

WEEK OF: _____

SPEECH & COMMUNICATION

SENSORY & O.T.

VESTIBULAR

TACTILE

ORAL MOTOR

MON

TUE

WED

THUR

FRI

SAT

SUN

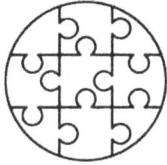

WEEK 12:

GOALS & PROGRESS
TRACKER

FINE MOTOR

VISUAL

AUDITORY

THIS WEEK'S CHALLENGES

THIS WEEK'S HIGHLIGHTS

SOCIAL SKILLS

FAVORITE MOMENT

WEEKLY APPOINTMENTS

WEEK OF:

MON

_____
_____
_____
_____
_____

TUE

_____
_____
_____
_____
_____

WED

_____
_____
_____
_____
_____

THU

_____
_____
_____
_____
_____

WEEKLY APPOINTMENTS

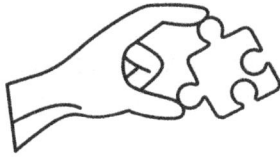

WEEK OF:

FRI

SAT

SUN

NOTES:

WEEKLY REFLECTION

Weekly Challenges

Weekly Accomplishments

Grateful For:

NOTES

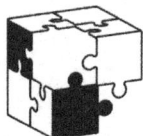

WEEK 13 ACTIVITIES:

MONDAY

TUESDAY

WEDNESDAY

THURSDAY

FRIDAY

SATURDAY

SUNDAY

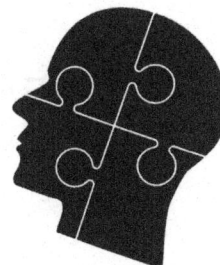

WEEK 13:

WEEK OF: _____

SPEECH & COMMUNICATION

SENSORY & O.T.

VESTIBULAR

TACTILE

ORAL MOTOR

MON	TUE	WED	THUR	FRI	SAT	SUN

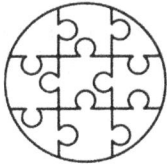

WEEK 13:

FINE MOTOR

VISUAL

AUDITORY

THIS WEEK'S CHALLENGES

THIS WEEK'S HIGHLIGHTS

SOCIAL SKILLS

FAVORITE MOMENT

WEEKLY APPOINTMENTS

WEEK OF:

MON

TUE

WED

THU

WEEKLY APPOINTMENTS

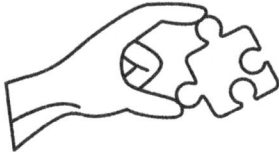

WEEK OF:

FRI

SAT

SUN

NOTES:

WEEKLY REFLECTION

Weekly Challenges

Weekly Accomplishments

Grateful For:

NOTES

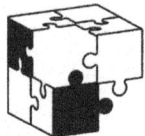

WEEK 14 ACTIVITIES:

MONDAY

TUESDAY

WEDNESDAY

THURSDAY

FRIDAY

SATURDAY

SUNDAY

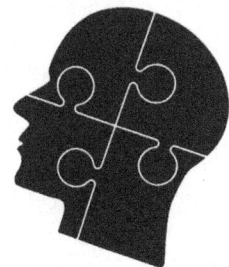

WEEK 14:

WEEK OF: _____

SPEECH & COMMUNICATION

SENSORY & O.T.

VESTIBULAR

TACTILE

ORAL MOTOR

GOALS & PROGRESS
TRACKER

MON

TUE

WED

THUR

FRI

SAT

SUN

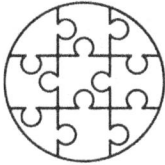

WEEK 14:

FINE MOTOR

VISUAL

AUDITORY

THIS WEEK'S CHALLENGES

THIS WEEK'S HIGHLIGHTS

SOCIAL SKILLS

FAVORITE MOMENT

WEEKLY APPOINTMENTS

WEEK OF:

MON

TUE

WED

THU

WEEKLY APPOINTMENTS

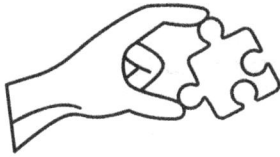

WEEK OF:

FRI

SAT

SUN

NOTES:

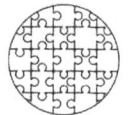

WEEKLY REFLECTION

Weekly Challenges

Weekly Accomplishments

Grateful For:

NOTES

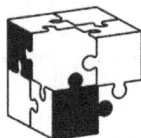

WEEK 15 ACTIVITIES:

MONDAY

TUESDAY

WEDNESDAY

THURSDAY

FRIDAY

SATURDAY

SUNDAY

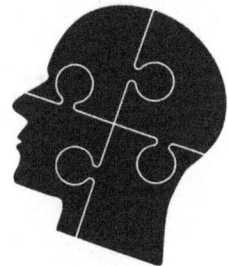

WEEK 15:

WEEK OF: _____

SPEECH & COMMUNICATION

SENSORY & O.T.

VESTIBULAR

TACTILE

ORAL MOTOR

MON

TUE

WED

THUR

FRI

SAT

SUN

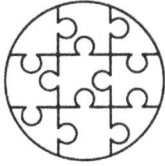

WEEK 15:

FINE MOTOR

VISUAL

AUDITORY

THIS WEEK'S CHALLENGES

THIS WEEK'S HIGHLIGHTS

SOCIAL SKILLS

FAVORITE MOMENT

WEEKLY APPOINTMENTS

WEEK OF:

MON

TUE

WED

THU

WEEKLY APPOINTMENTS

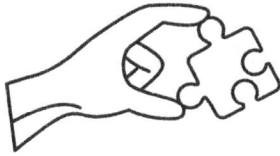

WEEK OF:

FRI

SAT

SUN

NOTES:

WEEKLY REFLECTION

Weekly Challenges

Weekly Accomplishments

Grateful For:

NOTES

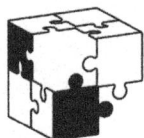

WEEK 16 ACTIVITIES:

MONDAY

TUESDAY

WEDNESDAY

THURSDAY

FRIDAY

SATURDAY

SUNDAY

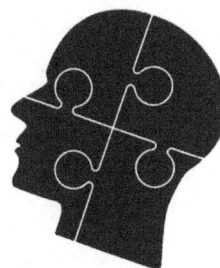

WEEK 16:

WEEK OF: _____

SPEECH & COMMUNICATION

SENSORY & O.T.

VESTIBULAR

TACTILE

ORAL MOTOR

MON

TUE

WED

THUR

FRI

SAT

SUN

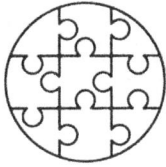

WEEK 16:

FINE MOTOR

VISUAL

AUDITORY

THIS WEEK'S CHALLENGES

SOCIAL SKILLS

THIS WEEK'S HIGHLIGHTS

FAVORITE MOMENT

WEEKLY APPOINTMENTS

WEEK OF:

MON

TUE

WED

THU

WEEKLY APPOINTMENTS

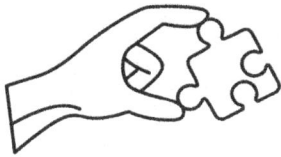

WEEK OF:

FRI

SAT

SUN

NOTES:

WEEKLY REFLECTION

Weekly Challenges

Weekly Accomplishments

Grateful For:

NOTES

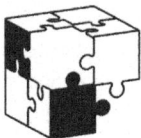

WEEK 17 ACTIVITIES:

MONDAY

TUESDAY

WEDNESDAY

THURSDAY

FRIDAY

SATURDAY

SUNDAY

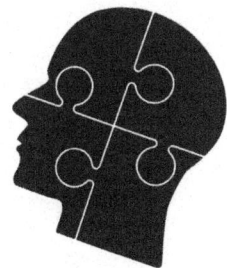

WEEK 17:

WEEK OF: _____

SPEECH & COMMUNICATION

SENSORY & O.T.

VESTIBULAR

TACTILE

ORAL MOTOR

MON

TUE

WED

THUR

FRI

SAT

SUN

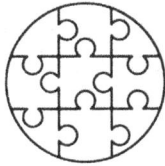

WEEK 17:

FINE MOTOR

VISUAL

AUDITORY

THIS WEEK'S CHALLENGES

THIS WEEK'S HIGHLIGHTS

SOCIAL SKILLS

FAVORITE MOMENT

WEEKLY APPOINTMENTS

WEEK OF:

MON

TUE

WED

THU

WEEKLY APPOINTMENTS

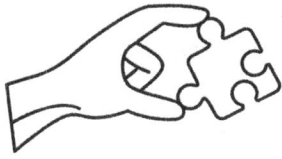

WEEK OF:

FRI

SAT

SUN

NOTES:

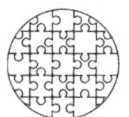

WEEKLY REFLECTION

Weekly Challenges

Weekly Accomplishments

Grateful For:

NOTES

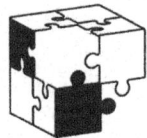

WEEK 18 ACTIVITIES:

MONDAY

TUESDAY

WEDNESDAY

THURSDAY

FRIDAY

SATURDAY

SUNDAY

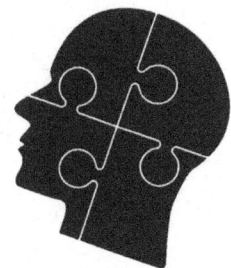

WEEK 18:

WEEK OF: _____

SPEECH & COMMUNICATION

SENSORY & O.T.

VESTIBULAR

TACTILE

ORAL MOTOR

| MON |
| TUE |
| WED |
| THUR |
| FRI |
| SAT |
| SUN |

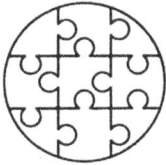

WEEK 18:

FINE MOTOR

VISUAL

AUDITORY

THIS WEEK'S CHALLENGES

THIS WEEK'S HIGHLIGHTS

SOCIAL SKILLS

FAVORITE MOMENT

WEEKLY APPOINTMENTS

WEEK OF:

MON

_____
_____
_____
_____
_____

TUE

_____
_____
_____
_____
_____

WED

_____
_____
_____
_____
_____

THU

_____
_____
_____
_____

WEEKLY APPOINTMENTS

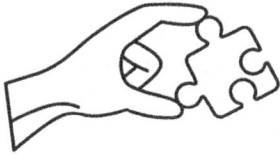

WEEK OF:

FRI

SAT

SUN

NOTES:

WEEKLY REFLECTION

Weekly Challenges

Weekly Accomplishments

Grateful For:

NOTES

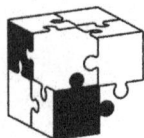

WEEK 19 ACTIVITIES:

MONDAY

TUESDAY

WEDNESDAY

THURSDAY

FRIDAY

SATURDAY

SUNDAY

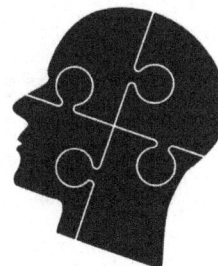

WEEK 19:

WEEK OF: _____

SPEECH & COMMUNICATION

SENSORY & O.T.

VESTIBULAR

TACTILE

ORAL MOTOR

	MON	TUE	WED	THUR	FRI	SAT	SUN

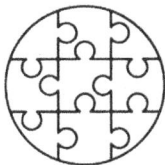

WEEK 19:

FINE MOTOR

VISUAL

AUDITORY

THIS WEEK'S CHALLENGES

THIS WEEK'S HIGHLIGHTS

SOCIAL SKILLS

FAVORITE MOMENT

WEEKLY APPOINTMENTS

WEEK OF:

MON

TUE

WED

THU

WEEKLY APPOINTMENTS

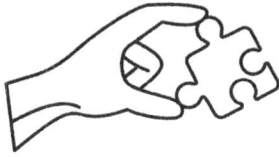

WEEK OF:

FRI

SAT

SUN

NOTES:

WEEKLY REFLECTION

Weekly Challenges

Weekly Accomplishments

Grateful For:

NOTES

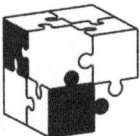

WEEK 20 ACTIVITIES:

MONDAY

TUESDAY

WEDNESDAY

THURSDAY

FRIDAY

SATURDAY

SUNDAY

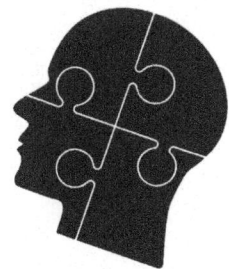

WEEK 20:

WEEK OF: _____

SPEECH & COMMUNICATION

SENSORY & O.T.

VESTIBULAR

TACTILE

ORAL MOTOR

MON

TUE

WED

THUR

FRI

SAT

SUN

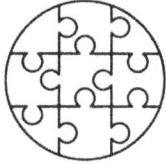

WEEK 20:

FINE MOTOR

VISUAL

AUDITORY

THIS WEEK'S CHALLENGES

THIS WEEK'S HIGHLIGHTS

SOCIAL SKILLS

FAVORITE MOMENT

WEEKLY APPOINTMENTS

WEEK OF:

MON

TUE

WED

THU

WEEKLY APPOINTMENTS

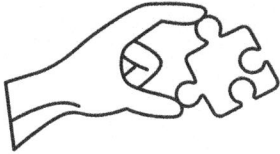

WEEK OF:

FRI

SAT

SUN

NOTES:

WEEKLY REFLECTION

Weekly Challenges

Weekly Accomplishments

Grateful For:

NOTES

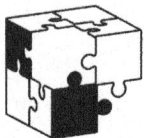

WEEK 21 ACTIVITIES:

MONDAY

TUESDAY

WEDNESDAY

THURSDAY

FRIDAY

SATURDAY

SUNDAY

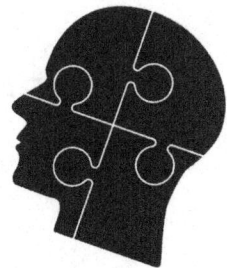

WEEK 21:

WEEK OF: _____

SPEECH & COMMUNICATION

SENSORY & O.T.

VESTIBULAR

TACTILE

ORAL MOTOR

	MON	TUE	WED	THUR	FRI	SAT	SUN

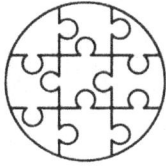

WEEK 21:

FINE MOTOR

VISUAL

AUDITORY

THIS WEEK'S CHALLENGES

THIS WEEK'S HIGHLIGHTS

SOCIAL SKILLS

FAVORITE MOMENT

WEEKLY APPOINTMENTS

WEEK OF:

MON

_____
_____
_____
_____
_____

TUE

_____
_____
_____
_____
_____

WED

_____
_____
_____
_____
_____

THU

_____
_____
_____
_____

WEEKLY APPOINTMENTS

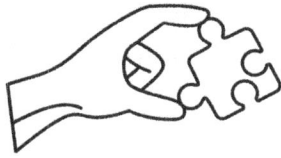

WEEK OF:

FRI

SAT

SUN

NOTES:

WEEKLY REFLECTION

Weekly Challenges

Weekly Accomplishments

Grateful For:

NOTES

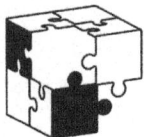

WEEK 22 ACTIVITIES:

MONDAY

TUESDAY

WEDNESDAY

THURSDAY

FRIDAY

SATURDAY

SUNDAY

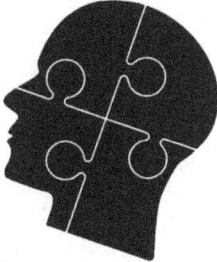

WEEK 22:

WEEK OF: _____

SPEECH & COMMUNICATION

SENSORY & O.T.

VESTIBULAR

TACTILE

ORAL MOTOR

MON

TUE

WED

THUR

FRI

SAT

SUN

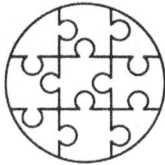

WEEK 22:

GOALS & PROGRESS
TRACKER

FINE MOTOR

VISUAL

AUDITORY

THIS WEEK'S CHALLENGES

SOCIAL SKILLS

THIS WEEK'S HIGHLIGHTS

FAVORITE MOMENT

WEEKLY APPOINTMENTS

WEEK OF:

MON

TUE

WED

THU

WEEKLY APPOINTMENTS

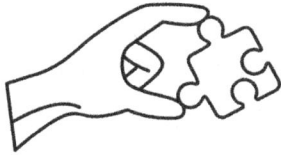

WEEK OF:

FRI

SAT

SUN

NOTES:

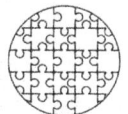

WEEKLY REFLECTION

Weekly Challenges

Weekly Accomplishments

Grateful For:

NOTES

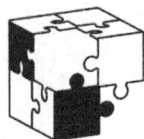

WEEK 23 ACTIVITIES:

MONDAY

TUESDAY

WEDNESDAY

THURSDAY

FRIDAY

SATURDAY

SUNDAY

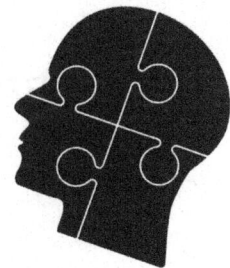

WEEK 23:

WEEK OF: _____

SPEECH & COMMUNICATION

SENSORY & O.T.

VESTIBULAR

TACTILE

ORAL MOTOR

MON

TUE

WED

THUR

FRI

SAT

SUN

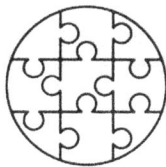

WEEK 23:

GOALS & PROGRESS
TRACKER

FINE MOTOR

VISUAL

AUDITORY

THIS WEEK'S CHALLENGES

SOCIAL SKILLS

THIS WEEK'S HIGHLIGHTS

FAVORITE MOMENT

WEEKLY APPOINTMENTS

WEEK OF:

MON

TUE

WED

THU

WEEKLY APPOINTMENTS

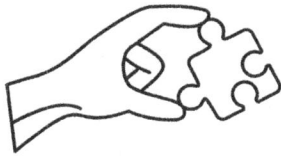

WEEK OF:

FRI

SAT

SUN

NOTES:

WEEKLY REFLECTION

Weekly Challenges

Weekly Accomplishments

Grateful For:

NOTES

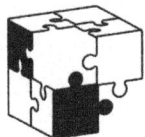

WEEK 24 ACTIVITIES:

MONDAY

TUESDAY

WEDNESDAY

THURSDAY

FRIDAY

SATURDAY

SUNDAY

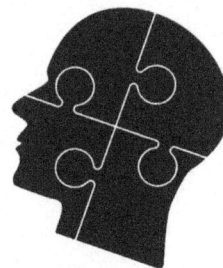

WEEK 24:

WEEK OF: _____

SPEECH & COMMUNICATION

SENSORY & O.T.

VESTIBULAR

TACTILE

ORAL MOTOR

MON

TUE

WED

THUR

FRI

SAT

SUN

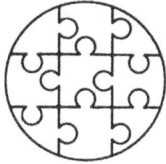

WEEK 24:

FINE MOTOR

VISUAL

AUDITORY

THIS WEEK'S CHALLENGES

THIS WEEK'S HIGHLIGHTS

SOCIAL SKILLS

FAVORITE MOMENT

WEEKLY APPOINTMENTS

WEEK OF:

MON

TUE

WED

THU

WEEKLY APPOINTMENTS

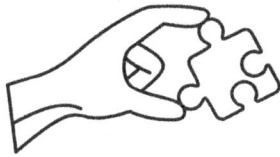

WEEK OF:

FRI

SAT

SUN

NOTES:

WEEKLY REFLECTION

Weekly Challenges

Weekly Accomplishments

Grateful For:

NOTES

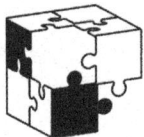

WE HOPE YOU LOVED USING YOUR PLANNER AND THAT IT HELPED YOU TO SCHEDULE AND STAY ON TRACK WITH YOUR CHILD'S OR STUDENT'S LEARNING AND DEVELOPMENT GOALS.

PLEASE TAKE A MOMENT TO LEAVE A REVIEW ON AMAZON TO SHOW YOUR LOVE :)

AND DON'T FORGET TO TAKE A PEEK AT SOME OF OUR OTHER COVER DESIGNS FOR YOUR NEXT 6 MONTH PLANNER

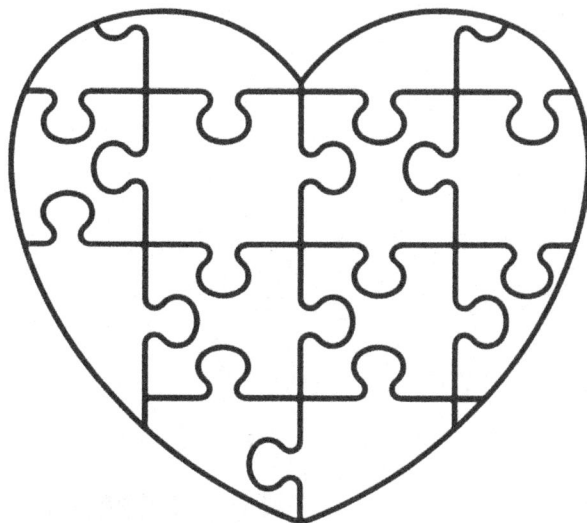

Made in the USA
Coppell, TX
12 January 2022